MINI HABITS FOR HAPPY KIDS

PROVEN PARENTING TIPS FOR POSITIVE DISCIPLINE AND IMPROVING KIDS' BEHAVIOUR

BUKKY EKINE-OGUNLANA

CONTENTS

Published by
TCEC Publishing
TCEC House

14-18 Ada Street, London Fields,
E8 4QU, England, Great Britain.

DEDICATION

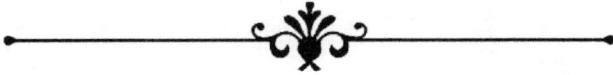

This book is dedicated to all the wonderful children all over the world who over the years have passed through the T.C.E.C 6-16 year's programme. Thank you for the opportunity to serve you and invest in your colourful and bright future.

INTRODUCTION

Research shows us that parenting a child with strong self-esteem is more effective than being authoritative. You want your child to listen, admire, and trust you instead of being scared.

All these things are easy to set as targets but challenging to accomplish. *How can you get the balance?*

The dynamics evolve as your child grows, and your views change, but your solution must be constant, intense, and caring. Help your child learn by practice, which helps develop trust and challenges. Calibrate your goals about what your child will do independently, whether you have a child who prefers to sleep through the night, a child who helps put away toys, or an older child who can settle disputes.

As a mom/dad, you can make a strong start of life for your children – they are nurtured, secured, and driven. Parenting is an independence mechanism that teaches your child. As your child grows and evolves, you will do a lot to support him/her. This guide will help you learn more about supportive parenting, stability, and wellness at any point in your child's life.

There is a myriad of techniques that are subject to debate between parents today. Parents find themselves going hoarse as they nag and shout and lecture their children frequently yet see no changes in their behaviour whatsoever. While every child is different, and this book will continue to reiterate that very fact, there are some tried and true strategies that parents can employ in order to improve their disciplining styles.

WHAT DO WE KNOW ABOUT DISCIPLINE?

The term *discipline* comes from a Latin word that means "to teach." As a parent, you are a teacher. How you discipline your kids will help them learn and frame their habits, even as they grow older in age.

For many parents growing up, discipline sometimes meant physical punishment or abuse. It could leave us feeling hurt, angry, and unjustly treated. Discipline is about teaching and guidance. It is a way to keep the kids safe as they grow older and discover more about life. To learn and get on with others, they need to learn how to control their emotions, desires, and actions. Without a doubt, discipline (and teaching the children appropriate ways to act) is one of the most challenging parenting elements.

While there are several different perspectives of how to discipline your child correctly, one concept that is consistent in these many different ideas is that the object of discipline is not merely to make your child behave in the next few minutes or even the same day but to direct your child through their developmental stages while teaching them valuable lessons and behaviours.

Warm but discipline out of love that stimulates the behaviour you want is the best way to train kids. A positive attitude is less challenging for children and makes parenting more fun. It takes time, but, in the long run, it is worth it. It uses love to teach life-long skills rather than fear, and it strengthens the bond with your child.

NURTURING YOUR CHILD

Nurturing is where you need to devote most of your time and effort. Kids learn best once they know they are valued and appreciated. Here are some ideas:

- Love your kids, no matter what they do – and show them you care.
- Listen to your children.
- When they act satisfactorily, praise them.
- Always expect the best of your children.
- Ensure they are safe, both physically and emotionally.
- Finally, be a good role model!

UNDERSTANDING CHILDREN'S BEHAVIOUR

Toddlers sometimes demonstrate their feeling in their behaviour. They are yet to learn the correct responses to say in every situation.

Parents might think the kid is 'naughty' or playing up when they are going through a lot in their mind.

It is essential to understand what influences the behaviour of your child. They will feel less desire to 'act out' or be 'naughty' if you communicate with what is bothering them.

It is easy to assume that you do not have the time to find out what is going on because life is so busy. However, the more time spent figuring out the actual cause of your child's behaviour would mean less time reacting to their misconduct.

LEARNING WHAT IS EXPECTED

Keep in mind that children are not born knowing how to act. They depend on you to teach them in ways that fit their understanding and skill. They need you to calmly and patiently show them what to do. Just as adults learn through practice, you may need to repeat a lesson several times until it becomes a mastery without your assistance.

That is why many parents get disappointed when the child does not get the point or does not break a bad habit immediately. In fact, you should expect this. You should expect that you will be drilling them with the proper behaviour before your child understands it and can master it without the need for your intervention.

After reading this book, please feel free to leave a review based on your findings and how useful the guide was to you. I would be incredibly thankful if you could take 60 seconds to write a brief review on Amazon, even if it's just a few sentences!

1

FORMS OF DISCIPLINE

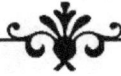

Disciplining children is a complicated feat that parents are faced with. Deciding on how to effectively manage your child's behaviour that suits both the child and the parents are intense conversations, but incredibly necessary for raising children. It is something parents have to reckon with reasonably early on, as children grow and are met with different social situations and deal with a myriad of new and complicated emotions. For most, acting out is a means of expressing these newly found emotions.

For parents, discipline is one of the many aspects of raising children that often bring about anxiety. Have you ever wondered how you can discipline your kids without being overly cruel or harsh? As it turns out, certain punishments can be a destructive discipline approach for your kids at whatever age they may be.

As parents, we must correct our kid as they grow older in age. Unfortunately, many parents overlook this, perhaps because they are scared to discipline the children. Of course, discipline is not the same as punishment – as many parents have mistaken it to be.

There are plenty of safe and appropriate methods that will educate your children on right from wrong. It is crucial to develop this compass within your children from an early age. It teaches them a myriad of things from responsibility to respect. As a parent, it is your duty to instil these crucial qualities, and while children are young, they will regularly test and push the boundaries.

So that you know, children will point the finger at their parents in the future if they get into trouble for wrong parenting. That is shameful, I would say.

Discipline involves teaching children according to rules to achieve the best behaviour that prepares them for the future. It invokes their brain and helps them function correctly in society. While discipline invokes the thinking mind, punishment impacts the emotional brain. Do you see why punishment could be destructive – especially for kids?

There are several forms of discipline that can effectively aid your children in mitigating their behaviours. Here are a few:

CALL A TIMEOUT

One of the most successful corrective methods available to parents of young children aged two years through elementary school years is timeout. The timeout solution is effective because it prevents the child from gaining attention that could unconsciously perpetuate improper behaviour. Like every other technique – when the kid misbehaves – you must use timeout unemotionally and regularly. Research shows that the timeout works effectively. However, you must understand how timeout works, how timeout is prevented, and what the parent does when the countdown is over.

Timeouts allow children to take a moment to reckon with the feelings that they are experiencing, as well as will enable the parent to take a moment amid the chaos to collect their own thoughts to react calmly and appropriately. Allowing your children a quiet moment to understand why they are being put in a timeout forces them to see why they were wrong and understand that there are consequences to poor behaviour. It's a method that is continuously implemented in households across the globe for its efficacy.

Understanding both your child's role and the role you play is crucial for the success of timeouts. You must prepare to speak to your child and talk them through why they are in this position in the first place. Listen to your children and recognize why they acted in such a way, to begin with. The key to the success of this method is listening and responding.

Some tips for parents on how to maximize timeout include:

- Introduce timeout by 24 months.
- Select the ideal location in the house where there is no access to electronic or digital tools.
- The timeout should last 1 min per year of the child's age to a maximum of 5 min.
- You should completely ignore a child who is in timeout.
- Do not forget to be the timekeeper.
- When the timeout is over, be friendly with them again and start new activities with them.

Similarly, you should avoid hurting your child's self-esteem by infusing shame, guilt, or a sense of loneliness. Ensuring that you are a reliable support system for your child begins here as you show them that despite their mistakes, you will still remain a constant force of guidance. Show them that while making mistakes can sometimes have consequences, the key is not to traumatize them and deny them of parental love.

Although timeout is an effective disciplinary technique, it may not necessarily eradicate the unwanted character. However, it can certainly lessen the frequency by teaching your children why it is wrong, and the consequences they face should they pursue this route. If you do not see any changes, get a consultation, and pray.

THE REASONING OR AWAY-FROM-THE-MOMENT DISCUSSIONS

Discipline requires both teaching good behaviour and modifying unwanted behaviour. In other words, kids need to know both what to do and what not to do. Generally, predicting and avoiding unwanted behaviour is more successful than punishing them for it. An away-from-the-moment conversation will help reduce negative behaviour by giving parents the chance to teach the child the desirable behaviour in advance. This technique is not suitable for use in children below the age of three to four years.

HERE ARE EFFECTIVE DISCIPLINE STRATEGIES:

Model good behaviour. If you want your child to behave appropriately, then let your child see you doing it first. How do you expect your child to behave well if you yourself do not show a model behaviour? You are your child's most excellent role model during these formative years. Reacting appropriately to the various stressors in your life will only reflect in your children.

Use positive discipline. Gone are the days were parents discipline their children with brooms or grounding them in their rooms, nor the threat of getting their gadgets. Today, many now advocate for positive discipline. Reward your child for good behaviour. That will undoubtedly lead to the retention of acceptable behaviour than punishing them for misbehaving.

Listen to them. If you catch your child misbehaving, talk to them, and listen to what they have to say. Find out the reason. Maybe your child is throwing a tantrum because your child is feeling jealous. Talk and listen to them instead of doling out the consequence of the behaviour immediately. Understand that your children are humans too. They experience incredibly complex emotions, especially at such a young age. Talking them through *why* they feel this way is a step in the correct direction to curbing misbehaviour.

Provide consequences. You must clearly explain to your child that there are consequences for every nasty action that they do. For example, you can tell your child that if they do not keep their play area tidy by returning their toys to where they should be after playing, you will store them away for an entire day. This sets them up for life to understand that this is something they will face increasingly as they age.

Be consistent. As a parent, do not waver in your discipline. You need to be consistent in how you deal with your child. You must show your child that you mean business every time they misbehave. If you have enforced a consequence for bad behaviour, make sure that you stick to it and not bail just after a few minutes because you feel pity for your child. Many parents find that this is the most challenging part. But understand that you are disciplining your child for their own good.

Apply redirection. There are cases where a child misbehaves because they are feeling bored. If that is the case for your child, redirect their energy to misbehave into doing something productive. For example, your 4-year old son is messing up his toys, and maybe he needs another thing to occupy him. Try giving him a colouring book and ask him to colour one page. Then check up on him after. Praise him for a good job and tell him to colour another page.

Revaluate age-appropriateness. Some disciplinary actions need to be age-appropriate. For example, you cannot really discipline a 6-year old boy the same way you discipline his 9-year old brother or sister. Keep in mind a child's age when disciplining them as certain punishments will have less efficacy, depending on what age or stage your child is at.

Avoid nagging, yelling, threatening, or punishing. As mentioned, gone are the days of threats and punishments. Countless studies have shown that punishments do not really help enforce good behaviour. It does the opposite instead. The same with nagging, yelling and threatening. These will only push the child to rebel and commit misbehaviour even more.

Many parents have struggled with finding a suitable disciplining style for their children, with many of them trying out different techniques and strategies before finding one that suited their child the best. While consistency is vital, finding an appropriate disciplining method that will have the most profound impact on your child's behaviour is more important. Don't be afraid to try different techniques. Some children respond well to timeouts, while some respond better to having privileges taken away. As your child continues to age, you may need to adapt to how you parent your child as well. The important thing is being receptive to your child's changing behaviours and growth in order to tailor the best methods to them in order for them to learn the correct actions correctly and safely. Know that it may take some time experimenting with different punishments. But once you have found what works best for both you and your child, stay consistent.

2

DISCIPLINE WITHOUT DAMAGE

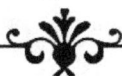

A child comes into the world with a blank mind: no ideas, philosophy, way to live or act. As they grow up, they depend on the family where they are raised. The parents (or siblings) then teach them and instil doctrines, values, discipline, and more.

Disciplining children is a universal thing that all parents are faced with. Regardless of your religion or culture, parents have the responsibility and duty of instilling the good qualities within their children. This is a universal understanding from the moment a child is born.

I grew up in a Christian home. My parents believed that there is no wisdom in the world except that which is from the scriptures – God's word. According to my parents, even philosophers derive their dexterity and wisdom from the word of God. So, they brought me up with the scriptures' views, and I am such kind of person now. Haha!

The word of God says, "Thy word oh Lord is forever and ever."

The bible is the only book in the world that stays true and shines in all situations. It guides and has answers to whatever life issues and questions anyone might have. And as it is with me, my parents instilled this knowledge in me from my toddler age to always turn to it whenever I need answers to life challenges. Of course, as a man, I cannot look elsewhere. Even now, I meditate regularly, reading and studying the scriptures – that is a habit I learned from my parent!

For me, as a Christian, my parents believed that there is no wisdom anywhere else, but in God's word, all philosophers only derive their philosophy from the word of God. So, the basis on which I was raised was from the book of books, which is from the word of God.

Thy word, oh Lord, is forever and ever. The bible is the only book in the whole world that is true. It has the right answers. If you know where to find it, I was instilled with the knowledge of God's word early so that I should not be looking for answers in a difficult situation later in life because I have been taught where to find answers, developing the habit of reading the bible regularly, meditating and studying the scriptures instils the right pattern into any child and once this has been done early, it is easier to navigate when the child finds him/herself in a difficult situation, the holy spirit will remind the child from what has been put inside.

For example, when Joshua was a kid, his memory was empty: he did not know anything or know life. His parents, however, filled his mind and brought him in the way of the Lord. He also went to the temple to learn from the teachers called "Rabbi." These precepts guided Joshua, and he was diligent in all his deeds, even till age 20. And God walked with him hence.

A child may come from a faulty culture or wrong philosophy. However, instilling the right habits will restore the child and make him readjust to the standard way of thinking or doing things. Discipline sets right and brings a child to his good senses.

Regardless of where a child comes from, understanding that there are societal standards of appropriate behaviour and responses to situations is crucial for their success. A parent's job is to instil these values, regardless of their beliefs. Parents have the freedom to do so; however, they please. Many choose to raise their children as their own parents have raised them. Some, with time and age, have chosen a different path. Despite technology and new parenting methods and trends that have come and gone, what has ultimately remained constant is that we are all human beings who need love as much as we need discipline. Instil this within your children so that they can continue to do the same as they eventually raise the next generation.

Whatever age your child is, between 0-12, keep in mind that you must be consistent in your discipline approach. The reason is if you are not serious, there is a tendency your kids will not take you seriously either.

You could have a blank paper to list ideas as they flow to your mind. After all, your kids will learn what they see you often do. With time, they tend to speak like you, dress like you, and walk like you.

Parents can be a possible climax to which children can arrive. My handwriting, for instance, was from my mum because she taught me how to write. Every child becomes like the parent or teacher who drills habits into them. All your child is emanating from you as a parent is your real you, which is very influential over your children!

INFANTS (BIRTH TO 12 MONTHS)

Infants need to drink, sleep, and play or communicate with others on a schedule. The schedule helps control autonomous functions and gives a sense of security and predictability. It does not overstimulate babies. As a parent, you should allow space for them to grow some resistance to anger and the capacity to self-soothe. You should not use discipline techniques such as timeout, spanking, or consequences.

EARLY TODDLERS (ONE YEAR TO TWO YEARS)

Toddlers are incredibly vocal with their emotions. When they are happy, they demonstrate extreme happiness. The same goes for the opposite emotions. As they are just barely grasping their emotions, toddlers often misbehave as a result of this.

It is common and natural in the early years of a child to play with physical objects and with the ability to exert their own will against others. Parental tolerance is accordingly recommended. To ensure the protection of the toddler, restrict aggression, and avoid disruptive behaviour. Cautioning the child with a "No" face or another very short verbal clarification ("No-hot") and guiding the child to an alternative activity works effectively. During such times, the parent should stay with the child to supervise and ensure that the behaviour does not recur. Moreover, to assure the child that you still love him or her regardless of whatever conduct.

Early toddlers are very vulnerable to feelings of abandonment. You should not keep them away from yourself in timeout. However, sometimes, you can become so upset with the child and may need to set a child's separation period.

Putting it into action: The toddler wants to play with a sharp object, for instance, a knife in the kitchen. Use simple words to try and express to them that they should not be playing with dangerous objects because they can cause harm. Collect the knife and ensure that you have placed it in a safe distance to avoid this from happening again and remove the child away from the environment. As children are incredibly young and small, their concept of time is different, and their attention span can be diverted quickly. Don't harp and linger on the subject for too long. Instead, redirect their attention to a more suitable activity such as playing a puzzle game or ball in another room.

LATE TODDLERS (TWO YEARS TO THREE YEARS)

The search continues for mastery, freedom, and self-assertion. At this age, toddlers are incredibly curious and seek to explore everything within their reach. As they test their newfound independence, your job is to establish the limits. The child's anger at the recognition of limits in such struggles contributes to outbursts of rage. Rage or willful defiance is not usually conveyed in this manner. The caregiver should be empathic, recognizing the importance of these manifestations. As a parent, you should continue to supervise, set boundaries and schedules simultaneously. Set reasonable expectations of the achievement capabilities of the toddler. Knowing how your child reacts helps reduce circumstances in which frustrations flare-up. Also, you should offer a concise verbal clarification and reassurance when the child regains control.

At this stage, children want to explore their independence and tantrums can follow when they are not given what they want in order to nip them at the bud, curb tantrums by leaning into your child's need for a sense of autonomy. Offer them choices, and often two is enough for kids at this age. For example, "What do you want to eat: some fruit or some cereal?"

Minimize meltdowns by being able to anticipate what triggers them. Children are creatures of habit, and you will quickly learn their reasons for having a tantrum often repeats itself. If your child gets upset when they are hungry, prepare ahead of time with several snacks. If they get cranky and overtired, be consistent with a sleep schedule that makes time for plenty of naps.

Your reaction to these meltdowns is just as important as how you deal with them. Keep your cool, no matter how loud or emotional your child gets. Your attention to them is already spurring them on and encouraging them to keep going. Calmly explain to them why behaving in such a way will not give them what they want and is not an appropriate response to any situation.

3

HABITS TO DRILL INTO KIDS EARLY

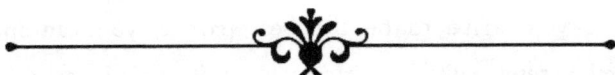

Most parents know full well that it is much less successful telling children what to do and how to behave than to show them what to do and how to do it. Teaching children a healthy habit early in life works better if parents themselves model their behaviours or behaviour.

Children search for encouragement from their parents, whether they are 3 or 13, so it is fantastic to drill these behaviours in children's early days.

We've all learned how successful people have similar characteristics and how they are the same across cultures and countries. But what if we told you that good parents have the same behaviours, too?

Everyone wants to know the secret of bringing up good kids. After all, no one wants a child that will not give them pride. Right?

There is something to consider before we go any further: **no one is perfect**.

While you strive to be the best parent, you can make mistakes repeatedly. You cannot deny it. This is something that parents face at some point or another. Just as much as they cannot be perfect, neither can their children be. Swallow this pill quickly, because for many parents, it can undoubtedly lead to a fractured and challenging relationship with their children that is fueled by resentment. Fortunately, if you take the right approach, your children will be placed on the road to potential success.

That said, now let us discuss practices to teach your children at the early stage.

CLEAN UP AFTER MEALS

Most children consume their food and sprint from the table afterwards.

They hope that their parents or brother would catch up. You do not want your child to have this bad habit. Instead, show them how to empty their dishes, rinse and place them in a dishwasher (if applicable).

When your child learns this pattern, it is likely to accompany her throughout her entire life, and it is also a transferable skill that will follow them for the rest of their lives, well into adulthood. Instilling a sense of responsibility within your children from these simple tasks will only help them in their future. Additionally, it applies to most good habits they develop throughout their lives.

MAKE THEIR BED

It is easy to wake up in the morning and disregard the bed, beelining for the toilet. Unfortunately, if you let this turn into a pattern, the remainder of your child's life will remain a concern (or maybe until they marry). Help them to straighten their bed, fold up the pyjamas, and set the pillows right. This act will not be perfect on the first day, but perfect is not what we want to achieve now but a habit to be cultivated even if it is not done correctly, but after some time, they will get the right routine.

A teacher once told the story about when Jesus rose from the grave, he folded up his cloth nicely, leaving us all an example to follow John 20:7. This story has helped the children in the class to be tidying their beds without reminders at home.

It will take your child some time to get into this schedule. If you do not let it slip, your kid will go by for a few weeks as part of their day.

Instilling this habit first thing in the morning encourages productivity from the start for your children. It encourages a sense of completing tasks the moment they wake and sets them up for success for the rest of their day as they have breakfast and go to school with a positive mindset. Making your bed might be seen as a frivolous task to many, but it can have incredibly effective psychological effects.

BE ON TIME (NO MATTER WHAT)

It is a concern many adults have, but you want to do whatever you can to secure it early.

You should inform your child how important it is to be on-time (unless it is a real emergency), regardless of what happens. It may not appear to be much stuff at a very early age, but that will change as your child hits school age. Each day, they will have to come to class on time.

This approach is one of the tougher behaviours to teach because some children do not understand time value. Yet, it gets easier for a child to adapt as they mature.

Taking up someone else's time is incredibly rude and tells the other person that you do not value their time. Teaching your children this from a young age sets them up for success as they enter school and eventually, the workforce.

HONESTY IS THE BEST POLICY

Is anything worse than lying? You do not want to have your kid into this poor habit early in life because it will take them into society and the workforce.

You should understand from an early age that integrity is the best strategy for your kids.

Indeed, your child may occasionally be lying, but you can never quit teaching. The more you speak about integrity, the more likely your child will take your advice. All kids come with a clean conscience, and lying will weaken their conscience and emotions if you do not help them.

For many kids, part of testing the boundaries is to lie to their parents and try to get away with it. But as the parent, spotting this may be easier than you might think. Part of raising children is that they grow more creative, and your job is to adapt to this. Your children won't have to lie to you if they can speak to you honestly and truthfully. If you seek to raise honest children, don't lie to them and accept that there will be shocking or scary things that they will share with you. But the worst thing for a parent to do is to judge their children harshly. Your first step is always to take a moment to process the information and then calmly offer advice, a solution, or simply a shoulder to cry on.

SAY "THANK YOU," "PLEASE," "SORRY"

Adults who do not know how to be courteous and respectful of others must have skipped this value at a young age.

Please have your kids in the habit of saying thank you and sorry (including related sentences).

Being gracious and respectful are some of the most basic expectations of a human being. Don't forget to instil these in your children as soon as they can form words. It is an essential requirement of humans to be grateful and apologetic when it is their time to be. Get your children used to thanking others for their time, for favours, or any act of kindness.

Tip: You must take this advice if you want your children to do this. If they see you disrespecting someone, such as your mom, they will start thinking it is all right, and it is not. Reflect the behaviours you expect your children to have.

READING

One of the most effective means of educating and valuing children is to teach. Parents should start reading to their children early every day or before they sleep. A strong reading base allows children to improve their language skills and communication skills in today's culture.

The One World Literacy Foundation says that reading skills are necessary because reading skills strengthen vocabulary, focus, discipline, memory, and develop self-confidence.

Instilling a love for books and learning from a young age will encourage a lifelong journey that is filled with education and creativity from books. When you read to your child, you are encouraging them to think beyond their environment and explore their imagination freely. Furthermore, there are several educational books that you can spend time reading with your children to teach them about more intense subjects that you may be nervous about broaching, such as racism and colourism. While the burden on a parents' shoulders is heavy to educate their children about everything in the world, reaching out to external resources like books are a great way to navigate through these topics.

"A person who does not read has no advantage over a person who cannot read."

— MARK TWAIN

STAYING ACTIVE

Another necessary behaviour is to be involved. Go out and play games and sports with your child. Cycle together and show them the value of fitness and being involved in a healthier life. Active children are less likely to have obesity or sleep disorders.

Furthermore, stop being a couch potato. Offer the kids a chance to participate and train school teams for a safe life.

Our health is something we take for granted, often before its too late. Teaching your children the importance of taking care of ourselves, while instilling a sense of self-love is incredibly complex and a huge responsibility that parents have to bear, but it is necessary. Many eating disorders stem from childhood habits that compound and develop in full force by adulthood. Curbing this by enforcing acceptable practices and a positive way of perceiving their own body is a strategy in combating this.

Remaining Positive

Children will quickly get down if things do not go as they want. To learn to be flexible when faced with losses or sacrificing something is a beneficial skill or pattern in early learning. The "strength of positive thought" creates self-esteem and contributes to a happier and productive future.

RESPECT

Children should learn to treat others early, including their elders, friends, and even animals. You see how your parents handle servers in restaurants or men who sort the garbage, and you benefit from these experiences. Being kind and respectful to others is a tradition that serves you when you get older.

Some people are bullying and shaming in today's online world, and children who have been polite from a young age will help break the loop.

Respect goes beyond merely treating your neighbours with kindness. Respecting oneself is just as important. Teaching your children to be kind to themselves in a world that will continuously have several hostile forces attacking them is crucial for raising confident and strong children. Allowing them to treat themselves with kindness and love is critical to them projecting the same attitude onto the people around them.

HONESTY

Say the facts once. Using errors and acknowledge the consequences. Integrity and dignity will continue with children all their life if their practices are practised early enough.

While understanding the nuances of lying, that will not harm others is something that your children will have to grapple with as they age, understanding that "honesty is the best policy" is the first step to raising healthy children—ensuring that your child has a good relationship with you is how to impart a trusting and honest relationship between parent and child. This way, you will always be aware of what your child is experiencing (particularly mentally) and be able to respond accordingly.

"Always do good. It will impress others and amaze others."

— MARK TWAIN

GRATEFULNESS

Children will often compare what their peers have and do not. Teach kids to be grateful for what they have in life and make them realize that there are still people who are less than they have. Learning early in life to count your blessings is a journey towards a quiet and peaceful life. It is a lesson that adults still face today, yet instilling this early on teaches your children to quickly face it and internalize the fact that this is the reality that they are faced with, where many people are better off than others, some seemingly so. This is where you attempt to educate your children on complicated topics like materialism and money in a simplified way. It can be extremely daunting, but even so much as trying already places you in the right direction.

FAMILY TOGETHERNESS

Provide as many reminders of the importance of the family as possible. Dinner together, exchange holidays with family members and allow them to be close to their relatives and friends wherever possible.

For many, we take our family for granted. We often assume that they will always be there, but this fantasy comes crashing down as we grapple with changing tides and the journey of life. Teaching your children to value family will only help them appreciate what they have at the moment. The concept of this is difficult for most kids to understand, especially depending on the age group. But spending time with your family and allowing them to experience your family members to the fullest and create beautiful memories is the best way for you to supply your children with a positive outlook on their family.

CLEANLINESS

A simple practice of brushing your teeth twice a day and learning how to flip holds your child's oral health in check. Brushing the teeth at night helps prevent bacteria from feasting on left pieces of food throughout the night. Flossing is incredibly important to manage plaque buildup and take care of your oral health. Showering or bathing and careful handwashing are healthy practices every day to establish early in life, for children. Hygiene is not always understood to be a top priority. When left to their own devices, children will get messy and dirty quickly. Teach your children to consistently practice healthy habits of hygiene in order to present themselves. Not only does this benefit them and the people around them, but it also helps their overall health.

FINAL THOUGHTS

This chapter is just a handful of the many routines that your young children can learn. When you have a plan in action, you need to commit to it if that is what it takes. Within a few days or weeks, some children develop healthy behaviours, while others battle for months. However, if you continue, things will quickly come together.

A last piece of advice. Travel with your children as much as possible to think about new cultures as well. Travelling exposes your children to the scope of how big the world is and offers them new perspectives and outlooks on life and the world. It encourages them to learn more about different environments that create more tolerant and empathetic children.

When you fly, the children get to see a more expansive world view, making them happier citizens. It gives them a greater sense of how much the universe has to offer.

4

DISCIPLINE OUT OF LOVE

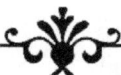

How can you teach your child consistency so that they can perform better at home and in public? Parents need their children to be safe, compassionate, respected, and willing to find their place worldwide and as well-behaved adults. Nobody needs to be credited with parenting a spoiled brat.

But often, these expectations seem to be miles away from the actual actions of your infant. Talk on obstacles to good behaviour, successful strategies of supervision, and aid in unsafe activity habits.

One thing that parents tend to forget is that they were children once too. Recall your own childhood and where you feel your own parents lacked or succeeded in when it came to raising you. Be reflective of yourself as you are your child's most outstanding role model.

ESTABLISH YOUR ROLE AS A PARENT

As a parent, you must help your child become self-sufficient, compassionate, and self-controlled. Families, teachers, churches, clinicians, health providers, and others can be beneficial. But parents remain the main burden for control.

The American Mental Health Association defines three parenting models – authoritarian, permissive, and authoritative. What is yours?

An authoritarian parent has reasonable goals and implications for his or her kids.

The influential parent requires versatility and mutual treatment of behavioural problems with the infant. Studies show that this is the most effective method of reproduction.

An oppressive parent has strong goals and ramifications but displays little love for his child. The parent might say things such as, "It is why I am the mum." This is a less successful type of parental education.

On the other hand, a permissive parent displays great love for his or her child but gives no discipline. This is a less successful type of parenthood.

Your children have to understand that while you are a trusty support system that will always be a constant force in their lives, they also have to be able to establish boundaries between parent and child. Finding that balance is often a challenge for many parents because as much as you want to be your child's best friend, you also cannot be a "yes man" which hinders their growth as a person.

DISCIPLINE TECHNIQUES

You can relate the type of unpleasant behaviour your child exhibits by their age, temperament, and, sometimes, your parenting style.

The American Academy of Pediatrics and the American Association of Child and Adolescent Psychiatry prescribe the following:

Good behaviour reward: The only way to inspire the child to proceed is to appreciate good behaviour. In other words, "Catch him as well." Compliment until your kid demonstrates the action that you were hoping they would do.

Social consequences: The child does something wrong, and you caused the child to feel the result. You do not have to "read." The kid cannot blame you for what happened. For example, if a child intentionally damages a toy, they do not get the toy.

Logical consequences: This approach is analogous to natural effects but explains the children's inappropriate actions. The effect is strongly connected to the behaviour. You warn your boy, for example, that if he does not clean up his toys, the toys will be confiscated for a week.

Removing privileges: There is often no rational or natural implications for incorrect actions — or you have little time to worry about it. In this case, a right can be revoked as a result of unacceptable actions. For example, if a middle schoolgirl does not finish her homework on time, her privileges can be taken away during the night. This technique of restraint works well if:

- In any manner, it connects to their actions
- The kid needs everything
- Taken as soon as possible after improper conduct (especially for young children)

Timeouts: Time outs work if you know what the kid did wrong or if the child's behaviour must be changed. Make sure you have a timeout place in advance. It needs to be calm, boring place-perhaps, not a bedroom or a risky area such as a bathroom (where the child will play). This disci-pline method will work on children while the infant is young enough to appreciate the intent of spending time-usually around two years and older. Time-outs also work well for younger children who view separation from their parents as a loss.

Why spanking and other forms of physical disci-pline do not work. Here is why:

- Spanking teaches kids that it is okay to hit when they are angry. You want to strive to teach your children anger management techniques, rather than more ways to lash out and negatively handle emotions.
- Spanking can physically abuse your kids or hurt them, which ends up having the effect of instilling fear in them, rather than building trust between the two of you.
- Instead of loving you or changing their misconduct, spanking makes them fearful and teaches them to avoid getting caught of their misdeeds. It fosters secrecy and ways to get around you.

TIPS FOR MAINTAINING DISCIPLINE

In all you do, ensure to direct your teaching to match the temperament of your kid. The secret to successful discipline is to consider your child, particularly his or her temperamental style, and use your discipline to help them reach their potential. However, it should not be your intention to let them him into doing something against their own will.

Say the punishment strategy. Discipline strategies are not meant to come "out of the blue," mainly when you try something new. When dealing with old enough children to grasp, explain the method during a scheduled conversation (not in the heat of the moment), why you are doing what you are doing, and what you intend it to achieve. Older children should be included in the option between incentives and consequences. Never act out of anger. Taking a breather to collect your thoughts and let your children simmer with what they have done is a positive thing for both parent and child.

Love your kids. Be compassionate. When you demonstrate respect for your child – significantly though your child is punished – your child will be more likely to respect you, your family members, and those in your own life. Apologize when you "lose it" or overreact in contempt. Act like them sometimes, if that works.

Be clear. Any strategy can fail if you do not systematically obey or apply implications. For example, if you claim your toys are out of limits for a week, take them away if the offending activity persists.

Avoid the lecture. While you may be incredibly disappointed by your child, save the long-winded lecture. Especially when they are younger, simply putting why you are disappointed by their actions and what they should do next time instead would suffice. Long-winded speeches often confuse children. You want to be clear and concise.

Do not crack the control. Do not give in by offering negative conduct in public events, such as a kid who throws a tangle while shopping. If you disagree with the demands of the kid, the tantrums will proceed. Know that the behaviour will pass and your child will be back to their happy selves, provided that you supply them with the right discipline.

Work to keep the priorities and methods intact over time. If more than one parent is responsible for the infant's discipline, please make sure that you compromise on the techniques.

It has not been done until it is done. Help your child come back to a suitable game.

Understand what is best for the growth of your child. Ensure that the kid fully knows what you wanted him or her to do before disciplining the infant. Parents often expect action which goes beyond the capacity of the child to obey. As with all essential life tips, behaviour also needs time for a frame-up.

Look for the "why" behind actions. When you see an unacceptable behaviour trend, part of the remedy is to search for "whys." For example, your child may be frustrated about something else or a friend leaving. Perhaps your child had a rough school day. Maybe your child is overwhelmed by family issues.

This does not explain the behaviour, but it allows you and your child to find ways to avoid it from repeatedly happening by seeking to explain why it happens.

Give time to relax and cool down. Sometimes, your child may do something that just really ticks you off. Instead of immediately reacting and scolding your child, give yourself a moment to cool down. Lie down and relax first. If you respond immediately to your anger, there is a greater chance that your anger will cloud your judgment.

Settle everything before bed. Try to settle matters before you go to bed. This will make sure that problems are dealt with as soon as possible. Just like we said earlier that brushing the teeth helps stop bacterial from feasting on little pieces of leftover food, in that same way, sorting things out before you sleep helps prevent anger from festering on the mind through the night. Going to sleep with everything resolved allows for the next day to be a fresh start of good behaviour. However, this does not apply to all problems because some need both parties to cool down and are best dealt with the morning after. Some issues are more complicated than others. But always bear in mind to try to resolve things before heading to sleep.

Create meaningful "heart-to-heart" moments. When you see your child often misbehaving, seat the child down, and talk to them about it. It is always better to settle issues with a good heart-to-heart talk, especially on sensitive issues. If you think that your child needs coaxing to let what they are feeling out, then you must initiate the conversation yourself. Be open and vulnerable to your child. This does not mean lay all of your own adult problems onto your children, but relate to them and express to them that perhaps you might have been frustrated today as well, but instead of taking out your anger by screaming and having a tantrum, you chose to deal with it calmly and rationally. Your children lead by example and having an adult that they can model their behaviour after. As your children age, perhaps the conversations can grow more serious and reflect the realities of the world. But in the meantime, while they are extremely young, don't be afraid to open up a little bit as well.

Use examples. When you try to discipline your child and teach them a lesson on something, try to use examples that they can relate to themselves. For example, if you want to teach your child the discipline of brushing their teeth every night, you can say, "if you don't brush your teeth before bed, you are allowing the germs to feast on your mouth, and you will lose your teeth." Sometimes a good bedtime story with discipline is a good trick.

KNOW WHEN AND WHERE TO GO FOR HELP

Give yourself a rest once you have the best discipline and style. There are days when nothing seems to fit. Maybe you had a bad day, too. It needs a lot of preparation and effort to develop skills for construction management. Be frank with yourself if you believe like you have made an error. Excuse your child and explain to the child how the next time you will expect to alter your answer.

Often you do not know what to do next. Parents are faced with a number of choices and the constant pressure of messing up that they panic and have moments of anxiety. Or you do not know how to alter anything more successful than what you are doing now. Perhaps you feel like you have hit a roadblock in your child's development and want more advice on how to proceed.

Whenever you have concerns about your child's actions and instruction, pray to God, and consult with your child's doctor. It could be time for a health specialist to support you whenever you see:

- A lack of regard or respect for other authorities such as guardians, teachers, and other adults in general.
- Actions that have been taught to be offensive or damaging, yet your children persist with this behaviour.
- Signs of despair, extreme sadness, lack of motivation long-term blueness, loneliness or lack of motivation. Sometimes the symptoms are not so clear and forward.
- Your child uses medications, drugs, or alcohol to treat depression or other life issues.
- Several family ties are complicated. Volatile relationships can affect your children negatively that they act out as a result in order to deal with the intense emotions they are experiencing.

FIVE GOLDEN RULES OF DISCIPLINE

Stand firm. We all hate confrontation, but if you do not obey the rules and repercussions you have created, your kids will not do so. It is that simple. So, do not waver in your decisions. If your kids see that you cannot hold on to the rules that you set yourself, they will not put importance on that rule and will eventually "slip up" and do it again. Or they may see it as a sign that you are not a strong authority figure in their life which allows them to act out and not afford you with the respect you deserve.

Pick your battles. Give little things little attention and big stuff much focus, and you are happy and calmer — and (bonus!) the kids are healthier, more relaxed, and stronger, too. You must remember that not every misbehaviour warrants your focus and vigilance. If you take notice of every little mistake that your child commits, you will end smothering your child. When children get too "smothered" with how you are, they tend to misbehave even more. So, give your child a break and focus only on their misbehaviours and mistakes when it is truly despicable. Remember that children are constantly testing the boundaries. For you to react strongly to every act of mischief and dole out punishment can take a toll on your own mental health as well.

Praise, do not punish. Continue to exercise mindfulness of positive feelings. Do not administer any punishment as that has already been proven to be a moot point. Instead, practice praising and positive feedback. In other words, your tone of voice, your actions, your vocabulary ought to sound good 80% of the time with your child. This act even works well as you cannot get it wrong. But although your voice is pleasant, do not forget to stay firm still. Most children want to be praised and be told that they are good and have made the right choices. Implement this in your parenting style because positive reinforcement is a force that really plays a profound impact on your child.

Set clear rules and expectations. A thoroughly chosen set of age-appropriate rules will make family life even simpler and cleaner, says Radcliffe. For instance, the "no cookies before dinner" rule avoids daily snacking claims before dinner. The "no machine after 10 p.m." law avoids a nighttime contention about the shutdown of the pc. You need to set up clear expectations of the rules with your kids. Do not provide room for misinterpretation as sometimes kids can exploit that to get their way. Maintain simplicity when setting the guidelines for your children. While expectations can be complex, it doesn't have to be for your kids.

Provide unconditional love. Yeah, it is a no-brainer, but kids need to know that every day, even though they have done something wrong, you love them. Show your kids that you love them despite the fact they misbehave systems. This will help your kids understand that you are fair to them and that what you are doing is for their own good. Despite the disciplinary consequences in place, make sure your children know that it comes from a place of love and care for them. Always make sure to spend time with your kids after the punishment to convey that all is forgiven. As you help your child grow and go through their own journey of life, you are a support system that will always provide them with the love they deserve.

5

CREATIVITY THINKING FOR KIDS

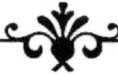

W ere you aware that you are creative? Even if you do not think your child is talented, God has made everyone exceptional and beautiful. God is the creator of all humans, and we are all made in his image and likeness. He encourages us all to use our imagination to make the world a better place. Moreover, we are a representation of him.

As humans, we often think of imagination as an innate trait or, sometimes, a learned skill. That is a very wrong concept: no one was ever-talented by birth. However, parents should encourage the imaginative thinking skills of their children at an early age. This can be instilled through a myriad of ways that may not be the most conventional either. Creativity stems from several methods and simply getting your child's brain thinking is already an act of exercising their creative skills.

Although you cannot promise that your child will become the next Picasso, you can give them a leg, giving them all the support, they need for imaginative thought. Activities such as arts, building blocks, and creative play will help the children develop their understanding and creativity.

Here are also various suggestions which will help parents encourage imaginative thinking and spending time with children.

EXPLORE SPACE

Learning about outdoor space often catches children's interest, so it can be a perfect way to inspire their creativity while allowing them the opportunity to venture into science lessons.

Furthermore, you can do many educational and imaginative things to stimulate your boy's fun activities for space.

Some of these exercises are very simple. You may encourage your child to use their imagination to tell you, for instance, what they believe the aliens are or ask them to tell a story about an astronaut who flew to the Moon.

You should also do creative exercises more deeply to inspire your child to learn about space. Solar panel paper mâché models are a perfect art activity for children, and Styrofoam balls will also render models.

Planetariums are another perfect way for your children to interact in nature. Planetariums also host fun movies and children's events to learn more about outdoor space. These outdoor excursions are an exciting way to spend time with your children. Science centers are another great way to learn about space, among a slew of other subjects like animals and chemistry. These centers are explicitly made to enrich your child's learning experience and go above and beyond to provide activities and learning opportunities with the number of experts and educators that are available at these centers.

These excursions apply for all ages, and parents often find themselves enjoying their time and learning a thing or two as well. While outings like these are not a common thing, they are a great way to treat your children and reward their good behaviour. They are also a great way to get out of the house and cater an outing specifically to your child that they will enjoy.

There are also plenty of online resources that are reliable and trustworthy for educating your children in a fun way.

For example, the NASA website is widely used by kids as it has an entire subsection dedicated to educating children with fun games, interactive videos and activities. Instead of spending their afternoons watching TV, perhaps take some time to sit together and explore these resources. There are several teacher-approved apps and websites that are recommended to enhance a child's learning further.

Encouraging your child's passion for open space through art and their creativity will help you build your home for your child. Space captures children and inspires them to try and visualize the wonder that exists outside of Earth, which is why it is so popular among children. The stars, planets and possibility of aliens capture children and exercises their brains to think outside of the box and outside the realm of possibilities. Studying space is a fantastic way to foster logic while also encouraging creativity in your children.

MAKE GIFTS

How do you let your children pick presents for their families as the holidays roll around?

Can you pick something tiny in the shop, or do you only have them in a package you have chosen?

If you want to do something else this year, your kids should make donations for others rather than buy something from the shop. Whereas the presents from shops bought by adults and youth are often well-thought-out, children's gifts often feel like an afterthought, unless handmade.

Creating presents for your children to send them to family members may be an ideal way for you to teach your children the value of offering presents. Unlike a small drink or card signature, it is a more intimate opportunity for the children to appreciate their friends and relatives.

Small beverages – such as bracelets or ornaments – are lovely and ideal creations for children of all ages, and you have much space in which to develop designs. You can paint wood ornamentations, learn how to braid friendship bracelets, or make adorable and unforgettable presents for your children by creating your snow globe kits.

When children grow older, they could choose to create advanced and customized products for the people they love. They can paint portraits of areas that your family loves, or they can carve, model, or craft more technical woodwork.

Gifts are a perfect way to foster ingenuity while allowing children to grow socially. Gift-giving is a great way to teach, especially younger children kindness and how to share their things. As your children age, they will love creating things that they are proud of that have a purpose for someone else.

They will want to share their talents and share the joy with those around them, which is why gift-giving is often met with such enthusiasm from children.

It is also a great way to spend time with your children. Arts and crafts are a fantastic way to get your child using their hands and tools while tapping into their tactile side to make a product that they have envisioned, planned for and executed.

MAKE TOY CRAFT KITS WITH YOUR KIDS

Toy craft kits are another perfect way to encourage creative ingenuity.

The kits are great opportunities to help your child practice their imagination while developing their fine motor skills. As an extra benefit, they can learn how to make things using their two hands.

Toy craft kits are available in all types. For younger children, you can do basic, easy-to-make, and personalize toys like pinwheels and tops. Easy and exciting science and craft kits are also available.

More complicated tasks might be appreciated for older children. You may want to make your own tea set or pound set, or you may want to make a model ship or train. You may get exciting chemistry kits or necessary devices for technologically inclined children.

Since there are so many toy craft kits online, you can easily find one that attracts your child, perfect for their ability level. There are also plenty of inexpensive options that can be found at variety shops. If these are also unavailable to you, purchasing inexpensive materials to come up with your own kit might take a little bit more effort, but will induce hours of entertainment and creativity for your child.

For more fun, make a family art project in which all your family members pitch. A birdhouse, a children's table, or other larger craft is one of the best ways to shape a family bond. These are great ways to get your children involved with nature and their outside environment as well. Remember that almost anything can be made into a child's playground. It's genuinely about how enforcing a positive attitude even towards the littlest things and encouraging your children to explore.

ENCOURAGE KIDS TO USE BUILDING TOYS

Design toys, such as blocks and Legos, can be fantastic opportunities for children to explore and expand their creativity.

You should give plenty of time for free playing with construction toys with your kids, but you should also challenge them to build something of interest to them. For example, if your 8-year-old likes cars, you could have a Lego car set and allow them to make a dream car.

You would have to consider a strategy that works to achieve what you want and set a realistic target. This principle helps your child practise their problem-solving skill while improvising to build the product of their dreams.

During free play with toys, your children can extend their imagination and play with objects. A little child might enjoy building a city with blocks to play with toys, and older children will enjoy building sets based on their favourite television and movie characters.

You should give your children plenty of space for fun, creative play with building toys, but you should also challenge them to keep them interested and aware. These obstacles should usually be opened to ensure that children continue to use their imagination. This style of toy is an ideal way to help your child grow their motor skills and spatial skills. They stimulate the imagination as they build simple to intricate shapes and also when they are demolishing their builds. Building toys encourage your children to think logically while also having a vision in mind that they are seeking to execute. This is a great skill that will accompany them as they age and enter school, and eventually, the workforce where problem-solving is crucial for every adult's life.

USE APPS, GAMES, AND GADGETS

Parents often ask the question, "Does technology limit innovation?" The answer is NO. Technology does not limit or affect a child's innovation in any way. Although spending too much time in front of the TV or some set of toys may be wrong.

However, using technology appropriately and in balance will improve children's innovative reasoning skills through software, games, and gadgets.

Many brain-boosting memories games and software out there are designed to help improve kids' memory in a fun and entertaining way. They help exercise your child's brain, improve concentration, enhance cognitive function, boost focus and attention.

Brain games will stimulate your child's thinking ability in unconventional ways to solve a problem. The benefits of brain games are numerous as they improve your child's memory and decision-making skills, as well as reaction control and their focus. Like physical exercise, the brain needs stimulation to improve upon analytical thinking, creativity, and problem-solving. The best part is that kids are likely to be open to the idea of a game as compared to, say, reading books. A brain workout for kids encourages a number of practical skills like planning, visual attention and employing some logic or math skills.

Similarly, language applications can help kids learn a second language. Learning a second language, especially at a young age, is extremely beneficial as children at this age are like sponges where they soak up new information far more quickly than an adult would. Encouraging a second language opens up a myriad of benefits as it exposes them to a new culture, new experiences and can significantly benefit them in the future. Learning languages also do not have to be intense practice unless they wish it. It can be as simple and as casual as simply watching cartoons in a different language or playing games in their target language.

Contrary to the assumptions of many parents, video games are not negative news for your child. If you choose to engage in age-appropriate games, they will improve your child's ability to believe and solve challenges creatively. You should also encourage your kids to play with various devices to relax and be curious about technology. This is also an excellent opportunity to educate your children on proper internet etiquette. Teach them about the dangers that lie outside of their bubble while also ensuring that parental locks are in place to manage their internet usage responsibly.

Gaming equipment, telescopes, and toy robots are beautiful tools that allow your children to explore technology to their imaginative thinking. Therefore, technology can be a fantastic way for children to stretch their imaginative powers, but parents can still be aware of how long their children are on the computer.

Although art apps or video games can help enhance fine motor skills and increase children's capacity to overcome challenges, they cannot replace real-life activities. While parents cannot focus on technology, it can be an excellent tool to build an exciting and creative atmosphere at home.

COOK WITH YOUR KIDS

It is undoubtedly overwhelming for children to cook. It is an opportunity to teach them a great life skill by improving their ability to solve problems creatively.

If your children are young, begin with essential recipes such as baked goods. It is easy to make muffins, cookies and loaf cakes like banana bread. For recipes of this nature, there aren't too many steps your young ones will need to adhere to. Plus, if you run out of milk or eggs, you will expose them to the idea of substitution and different techniques and methods for problem-solving in the kitchen. Exposing them to the kitchen from a young age ensures that they are not intimidated by the kitchen as they age and will be motivated to try cooking when they reach older ages.

As your children grow older, you could expose them to complicated recipes that require more abilities to prepare. For instance, you can begin with Cottage Pie then to a more complex Boeuf Bourguignon recipe. Encourage them to try new foods and find recipes that excite them. Allow them to take the reins and offer minimal help unless asked. Give your children the chance to spread their wings and flourish in new territory. While mistakes can happen, guide them to make sure they are practising safe habits.

Although it will take longer for your children to eat in the kitchen, watching them learn and grow up would be worth-while. Besides, cooking is an experience that you will enjoy with them even though they might be adults at that stage.

Getting your children in the kitchen is a great way to encourage independence and teach them skills that are important for the future. If your children are picky eaters, in particular, getting them involved with cooking and baking can show them to be unafraid of new foods and flavours. It can get them excited to eat as they have a hand in the process of creating the final product. You will not only offer your children an invaluable skill to use later in life, but it will also help develop their capacity to think creatively, solve challenges, and handle resources.

MAKE ART WITH YOUR KIDS

Making art for your children is one of the easiest ways of turning your home into a fun, artistic space.

Kunst is an effective way for children to express themselves and develop their artistic skills. It improves your motor skills and encourages you to expand your creativity.

You should still ensure that you have art supplies in your house. You do not have to buy a Hobby Lobby, but some pencils, Play-Doh, and coloured paper will help inspire your children to make use of their imagination regularly. These tools are inexpensive but can inspire your children to create pictures and projects that allow them to express their creative side. Fostering this habit will enable them to think outside of the box and come up with their own original ideas.

You can also create art projects for your baby. While you may not be an artist, you should indeed teach your child basic crafts such as making flowers from tissues and pipes or making festive paper chains.

Signing up your children for art lessons with your child is another beautiful way to communicate with your child while art is being made. Parent-kid pottery lessons are a disorderly yet enjoyable way to communicate and build with your kids, and you should use these classes as a chance to practice together if you are not the most skilled artist.

You will let them develop their imagination by making art with your children while improving their ability to articulate themselves and travel carefully.

TEACH THEM HOW TO PLAY MUSIC

Another perfect way to inspire innovation at home is to play music with your children. Music is a well-loved extracurricular that parents all around the world encourage their children to pursue. It fosters a discipline and a sense of responsibility. It also increases memory skills and improves their coordination. Having an education in music teaches your children to persevere and as they meet the goals that they have set for themselves, gives them a sense of achievement. It is also another effective way to nurture self-expression.

If your child is an only child, you can assist with this by giving them necessary instruments like kids' keyboards and drums, and you can even enrol them in music lessons targeted at children.

As your children step closer to adulthood, you should teach them the fundamentals or enrol them in beginner lessons for simple instruments like the piano.

Children from primary school will have plenty of chances to participate in music when they grow older. Schools will also have music lessons for children singing and playing a recorder, and your children should enter music clubs.

Your kids will also be part of the school band, chorus, or orchestra if they want to play different instruments and practice music.

Even when your kid is not close to nearby Mozart, you must teach them how to play music to learn about their talent and cultivate their love for good music.

MAKE A PHOTO BOOTH

Taking a photo booth is a perfect way to dress up, offer photography to girls, and at the same time, make invaluable memories.

You can begin by collecting old clothing, fun costumes, and fascinating tips around your home by making a photo booth for your children. While you should still purchase things that your children like, you should be sure to find many dress-ups at home.

You can visit the nearest thrift store if you need a few additional supplies. Thrift shops are often packed with fun-and cheap-items to wear while your children are dressed.

Next, you can build a picture area for your children. You can clear a specific wall or hang a sheet for a lovely backdrop, and you can catch some lamps to boost lighting in any room.

Then dress up and snap away from your children! If your children are old enough, you can show them how to use the camera, and you can also involve them in the setup.

You will have a set of pictures at the end of the picture, put in your scrapbooks, and save them for when they are older, and your kids will have fun.

Creating a photo booth is the best place for your children to make lasting memories and be imaginative.

Some children might prefer to be on the other side of the camera, so always consider the flipside as well. In this case, teaching your children the essential functions of a camera and then allowing them to use their creativity and imagination to take pictures as they see fit is a great way to foster another hobby from a young age.

GO ON CREATIVE "MINI FIELD TRIPS"

Small businesses in areas that foster innovation will help connect your child to fresh and exciting experiences. Encourage outings with your children to explore your local areas. Go on walks and explore the nature that surrounds you. This way, your child becomes more acclimated with spending time outside, gets plenty of fresh air and exercise, and is more in tune with nature, which has its own way of relaxing a person.

Museums are a convenient and cheap way to inspire innovative thought. Children's museums also have a wide range of displays suitable for children and are packed with enjoyable, hands-on experiences that allow your child to experience the world around them.

Other museums, such as art museums or museums of natural history, are also excellent opportunities for youngsters. Although your children should be old enough to grasp the museum's etiquette, these types of museums are perfect examples of teaching your child and stimulating your mind.

Theatre shows are just another fun experience when encouraging your children's artistic climate. Age-appropriate plays and musicals are great opportunities to get the children into theatre, and many children's theatres offer children's acting lessons.

The library is another excellent place for children as there are often sections dedicated for children that feature books, computers and reading corners explicitly designed for entertaining and educating your children. For a bit of quiet time, consider going to the library where your children can pick up their favourite book. If your child has a little bit more energy and is unable to focus, read-alongs are often planned events at libraries that are free to join and a fun way to spend your child's afternoon.

You may also participate in concerts and symphonies to improve your child's music's passion and enjoyment. If it is classical music or a successful singer, your child will grow their talent at live music events. This is a great way also to show your children how music can be transformed in a concert environment. Many musicians and artists have been created in these spaces, where at a young age, they witnessed performances and felt inspired to pursue the arts in the same way.

You can also check at local activities and see if your children can be involved in nearby exhibitions or as speakers. Excellent theatre and history can be enjoyed for your kids at events such as Shakespeare in the park and Renaissance events. Exhibitions on Ancient Egypt or space shuttles can be fantastic opportunities for them.

It becomes apparent that there are hundreds of ways to improve children's imagination, and most of them do not take time. When considering an after-school service, parents should not even have to assist in the curriculum process. Therefore, never fail to inspire children to improve their creative ability, as innovation in the modern world is key.

ORGANIZE STUFF AT HOME WITH YOUR KIDS

You do not have to go far to build a relationship with your kids and enhance their creativity as well. You can do that just in the comfort of your own home.

You can select a specific day as your "home decluttering day." It will be a day where you spend time with your kids, decluttering your home, and organizing stuff. Give your kids the chance to decide how they can help you keep things organized. Maybe one of your kids will decide on a labelling system for the boxes with the stuff. Perhaps one will be able to make DIY containers. Let your kids' imaginations run free in their organizing.

This will not only instil the habit of keeping things in order in your kids, but it will also help them develop their critical thinking and creativity in solving problems like storing stuff in a small space, lack of storage containers, recycling things, and more.

LET YOUR KIDS ORGANIZE A YARD SALE

After your decluttering activity with your kids, you can help them organize a yard sale for the excess stuff. This is especially helpful for kids aged nine and above.

You can let your kids help in placing price tags on the items. You can even let your kids help in talking to customers who will buy stuff from your yard sale. Just make sure to supervise them well. It's a sure way to teach your children the value of money as well as some incredibly basic methods for managing funds.

This will help your kids feel a sense of accomplishment. Do not forget to praise them for a job well done as well. Even if you were not able to sell everything, the fact that your kids were able to start up the yard sale should be a great learning opportunity for them already. It will help them let out their ingenuity and let them learn the ropes of business early as well.

PRAYER:

Thank you, Lord, for making us in your image. Allow us to use your gifts and imagination to make the world a better place. In the name of Jesus, Amen.

6

THE RIGHT DISCIPLINE FOR KIDS

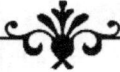

The discipline techniques you choose will depend on the type of unacceptable behaviour that your child shows, your child's age, your child's personality, and your parenting method. It can be extremely beneficial using the following techniques.

An adult with more than one child or child care provider will agree that what succeeds with one child's parenting strategy cannot work for another. Variations in how children respond to punishment may raise a risk that their strategy is not compatible with parents.

Consequently, it is not shocking that more than one-third of parents do not believe their parenting strategies perform well, based on a survey conducted in 2007 by 2,134 parents of children aged 2 to 11.

Luckily, child psychologists have demonstrated that constructive and successful parenting methods for parents have shared foundations. Here are a few strategies to try:

CONSISTENCY IS KEY

As each person has a different parenting/caregiver style, all supervision should be apparent all the time. Help to establish clear guidelines and methods as well as expectations and incentives every day. Changes or contradictions can be challenging for youngsters, and limitations or limitations can be checked to see how far they can go for different adults. Consistency is essential for predictability in parenting. Parents become predictable to their children because their responses and outcomes are consistent. Your child will foresee how they will respond to such circumstances.

So, be consistent with your words, actions, and decisions when it comes to disciplining your child. If you are inconsistent yourself, how will you expect your child to follow the rules that you set consistently?

SEEK OUT THE 'WHY' OF MISBEHAVIOUR

If your child throws a cup and its substance spills, you would think that is unexpected, right? However, if you have time to look at the "why" of the behaviour instead of just the action itself, the child's concern (at least in this instance) might be more apparent. Whether you decide that the strokes were trapped, you might predict a result other than whether they threw it because they did not want milk for a drink. Sometimes, it could be that they were furious about something else, and that was the best way to react. Parents will always subject their child to a more acceptable action and a fair judgment by understanding their behaviour's root cause.

Disciplining your child is essential, this is something most parents are aware of. But most of the time, there is a root cause for poor behaviour that parents may neglect to examine. They may not see a way out as they feel completely in over their heads with trying to deal and manage their child's behaviour effectively. It can be incredibly overwhelming for parents. However, understand that part of the job is not just to deal with the aftereffects of poor behaviour. A big part of successful parenting is receptive to the changes in your child, especially emotionally.

So, when next you see your child acting out or doing unexpected behaviour, take time to talk to your child. Find out what is wrong instead of simply deeming it punishable. That way, you will find the "why" behind your child's behaviour and nip it in the bud, instead of allowing it to continue to fester and flourish into several other problems down the line. While parents are humans too and are not all-knowing, keeping this in mind while you discipline your children is helpful.

AVOID POWER STRUGGLES

Choose your challenges wisely – but if you have identified a fight, a parent/adult can prevail most of the time. Fix only those critical (security is still a big fight) and let other things go. But if an issue is significant, the parents should try to avoid giving in to their child, even though this is "just once." If you do, then any time this issue emerges, your child may realize that you will only change your thoughts again and groom.

So, know when to give in and when to force your way. If you see that the issue is not really that big to fuss about, then give your child some leeway. But if the problem is serious, then you absolutely cannot loosen your hold on the rules. Instead, maintain the strictness and enforce it even more.

Your child has to understand that you are the adult in the relationship and bear the responsibility of ensuring that they adopt the right habits and behaviours. For them, it means that they have to respect the boundaries that are in place between parents and children. There is a fine balance here that needs to be struck where your children understand that you love them unconditionally, but there will be consequences to poor behaviour.

EMPHASIZE AND PRAISE GOOD BEHAVIOUR

If your child's wrongdoing does not cause any harm, like tanning, whining, or other misconduct, you may opt to disregard with it. In such cases, an appropriate constructive corrective strategy may include celebrating the right actions and rewarding them with embraces, high fifths, or fun events such as a visit to the park. While it is much easier said than done to ignore a crying kid, they will ultimately learn to equate good behaviour with positive reinforcement and recognition while learning that their poor actions will not get them anything.

So, do not be stingy with your praises. If you know that your child has done well in showing good behaviour, then praise your child for it. Children thrive on praise. You don't always have to implement rewards, but simply offering kind words and praise does plenty to encourage and even inspire your children to pursue good behaviour. Remember that praises gain better results than punishment and harsh words.

KEEP YOUR COOL

Kids are fascinated by what an adult does. They are always absorbing your actions. However, they might sometimes find these activities confusing.

Talk to your child to stay calm and reassure them if they find themselves in such a state of turbulence. Teach them to remain calm and relaxed in whatever situation, even unpleasant ones. Knowing how to stay calm and cool is an essential trait to learn and must show your kids, as their immediate reaction to stressors can often be explosive. By no means are we encouraging children to bottle up their feelings. However, parents should teach their children that responding to situations calmly in order to self-regulate and manage anger is more beneficial. Forgoing this can bring about several problems for your child's future, as they are met with increasingly challenging social situations. It can cause a lot of damage and be a deterrent for future relationships your child will have with other people.

As you instil being calm to your kids, you must also exhibit this trait, especially in front of them. Remember that children learn better when they have someone to refer to the trait. So, if you want your children to grow calm and know how to keep their cool, you better do it yourself first.

SEEK OUT DISCIPLINE SUPPORTERS

Whenever someone else watches your child, make sure that you express your discipline method and urge the guardian to follow a similar approach. Likewise, if you do not believe in a specific solution, please tell a babysitter or an early childhood teacher of this too. Take the opportunity to inquire about their training techniques to look for a potential daycare or nursery. Parents will find that the findings become more successful if they align their methodology to childcare approaches. The explanation may be that children respond to behavioural tactics used by their peers.

When someone else takes the helm of disciplining your child, even for just a day, you must make sure that whoever it is, they know your discipline style. For example, if you do not allow your child to eat ice cream past 9: 00 PM, then the baby sitter should adhere to this rule as well, no matter how your child begs them to consider.

EDUCATE YOURSELF ON PARENTING AND DISCIPLINE STYLES

There are various varieties of parental methods and disciplinary techniques. Training in different ideas will allow you to be more knowledgeable and regulated when deciding how to respond to your child's circumstance. If you chose optimistic, boundary-based, gentle, or other styles, it is essential to understand what every style is and choose what best suits your culture.

You need to brush up on these parenting styles so you could shape a style of your own that will best fit your children. Try to listen to how other parents deal with their children and pick up what you think will work for you. Doing research and reading parenting books are also great resources where you can learn.

While there can be so many tips and tricks out there that parents swear by, finding one that suits yourself and your child can be a gargantuan task. But part of the process is trusting yourself to know what comes naturally to you as ultimately, you know yourself and your children the best.

HEALTHY DISCIPLINE STRATEGIES THAT WORK

The AAP recommends positive discipline strategies, which effectively educate and prevent children from harming their actions while promoting healthy growth. This includes the following:

- Show and tell. Teach kids right from wrong with steady words and deeds. You want to see model patterns in your children.

- Set restrictions. Have consistent and straightforward guidelines that your kids should obey. Make sure to clarify these laws in age-appropriate terminology.

- Give results. Explain the consequences politely and firmly if they do not act. For example, remind him/her that you are going to put it away for the rest of the day if he/she does not choose his/her toys. Be able to step up directly. Do not give in for a few minutes by handing them up. But please, never take anything your child wants like a meal away.

- Hear them out. Listening is important. It is important. Enable your child to complete the story before solving the dilemma. Look for occasions when wrongdoing has a trend. Speak about this with your kid; do not just offer implications.

- Give them your attention. Attention is an essential weapon for successful discipline — to improve positive conduct and deter others. Note, both children want the love of their parents.

- Catch them good. Children deserve to know when they are doing something wrong and when they are doing something right. Note positive conduct and show it, enjoy the performance and successful attempts. Be descriptive ("wow, you've done a nice job putting the toy away!"). Be precise.

- Know when not to speak. If your kid does not do anything dangerous and thinks about acceptable behaviour, avoiding negative behaviour may be a successful way to prevent it. Misconduct will also show children the normal results of their behaviour.

- Be prepared for difficulties. Hop for whenever your child has problems acting. Prepare them and the way you expect them to behave.

- Bad actions reverse. Often children's misbehaviour is usually due to whether they are lonely or because they do not know anything better. Find out what your child would love to do and set them right in.

- Call timeout. A pause can be beneficial if a particular law is violated. This method works well to warn kids if they do not quit, warning them of what they have DONE wrong. You should only say "go back and forth whenever you are comfortable and in charge," which can help the child develop and improve self-management skills, which works well for the elderly and teenagers.

RESPONDING TO TANTRUMS

When a child is tired, starving, irritated, or frustrated, tantrums usually result. Maybe your child would keep her fists clenched, close her eyes, and scream. He may kick, throw himself to the floor, and create a scene around it.

Make efforts to prevent tantrums from happening. Ensure your child gets enough sleep. Do not take them out when they are tired or hungry. If you must do, bring along healthy kids, food, toys, or books to keep your child engaged throughout the outing.

Why are tantrums so common at this age?

- Kids are curious and explore all they can to find answers to what amuses them.
- Children are faced with new emotions and a natural response to convey some of these complicated emotions and display their discomfort is through a tantrum.
- Because they might not express themselves adequately, they might turn out to become angry.
- When children are hungry or frustrated, they often react with unpleasant emotions or behaviour.

Keep in mind that tantrums are normal among kids. So, leave them to experience this if they are not hurting themselves or someone else.

What can you do as a parent?

Try Distraction: distracting your child from their interest in something else works in your response to a tantrum as a parent.

TIPS FOR APPLYING CONSEQUENCES

- Apply consequences almost immediately.
- Avoid getting into arguments with your kids during the correction process.
- Make the consequences short. For instance, the timeout should be for just a minute to a maximum of 5 minutes (depending on the child's age).
- Be serious when you correct the kids but do not yell at them.
- Explain to them why they are being punished for their behaviour. They should be able to explain back to you why they acted in such a way and that it is wrong.
- Always follow consequences with love and care.

BELOW ARE SOME EXCERPTS.

- Avoid nagging and making threats without consequences. The latter may even encourage undesired behaviour.
- Apply rules steadily.
- Ignore irrelevant behaviour such as swinging legs while sitting.
- Set achievable limits, maybe every week.
- State acceptable and right behaviour that is workable.
- Prioritize rules. Giving safety top priority, then to correct actions that damage individuals and property, and then to conducts such as temper tantrums and disruption. You may focus on two or three rules for a start.
- Accept mistakes bound to their age limit. For instance, they were accidentally spilling water on the floor.
- Understand their temperament and raise them accordingly.

7

PROBLEM HANDLING FOR CHILDREN

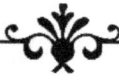

I f your kid cannot find his math homework or forgets his lunch, the secret to helping him navigate his life is strong problem-solving skills.

In a 2010 report released in Behaviour Science and Treatment, the risk of depression and suicide was greater for children lacking problem-solving skills.

The researchers have found that teaching a child problem-solving skill would enhance their emotional health.

You will continue to teach simple problems during preschool, which will help your child develop their high school skills and beyond.

REASONS KIDS NEED PROBLEM-SOLVING MINDSET

Children face a host of challenges every day, from school issues to athletics challenges. However, a few of them have a method to fix these issues.

Instead of investing their resources into fixing the problem, they will spend time ignoring the problem. Therefore, so many children fall behind in school or why they fail to keep friends.

Some children who lack the desire to overcome difficulties do not understand their decisions. A child can strike a peer who cuts in line in front of him because he does not know what else he should do.

If he is tinkered, he may go out of class because he cannot think of any better way to stop it. These impulsive actions will, in the long-term, cause much greater problems.

TEACH KIDS HOW TO EVALUATE THE PROBLEM

Children who feel confused or helpless will sometimes not want to fix a dilemma. However, they will be secure in their ability to solve a crisis when you give them a simple method or guide to solve problems.

Here are the steps to solve the problem:

- Define the problem. Simply mentioning the issue will make a significant impact on children who feel lost. Support your child to state the case, for example, "You have no one with whom to play in recess," or "You do not know whether you can take advanced math's."
- Create five potential alternatives at least It should be emphasized that not all proposals ought to be successful at concepts (at least not at present). Support your child to develop strategies if they fail to generate ideas. Such a dumb explanation or a far-fetched idea is conceivable. The key is to make him see that he can discover several different alternative options with a little imagination.
- Identify the benefits and disadvantages of each approach. Help your child consider potential positive and negative outcomes with any possible solution it has found.
- Choose a solution. After the future good and bad effects have been measured, motivate your child to find a solution.
- Try it out. Find a solution to see what is going on. If it does not fit, he/she can still find a different approach in phase 2 of the list he/she created.

There are unavoidable bumps, potholes, and unsafe zones in addition to all the valuable moments and memorable memories.

It may feel a little like a ride down a bumpy path to help your child solve problems, encounter dead-end after dead-end, and lose sight of the target.

You want your child to feel like you are working together to fix issues and not just lecturing and wiping them up!

TIPS FOR PROBLEM-SOLVING WITH YOUR CHILD

Here, then, are some tips to manoeuvre through the problem-solving minefield with your child:

1. Try not to play the role of "Mr./Mrs. Fix-It".

Sometimes, children are disappointed by a solution that is not correct now with their unique situation. So, give your child autonomy and a chance to work things out for him/herself. Remember that experiencing the process of decision-making and looking for solutions for problems can be a better lesson for your child, rather than fixing the problem yourself and telling your child about it.

2. Help them to find their answers and solutions.

As parents, you want to do all right, of course, but in the end, you want to encourage problem-solving in your girl/boy.

By encouraging your child to find his/her ideas and responses, you motivate the child to feel empowered and deal with the skills. As your child feels empowered to solve the issues, he/she is dealing with, and it will breed even more sense of achievement. It is a cycle. So, you must be a pillar of support and be a guide for your child as he/she tries to solve problems.

3. Teach your child how they can "survive" difficult or unpleasant feelings.

Although they may not feel confident about frustration, rage, sadness, and remorse yet, your child needs to learn to control these emotions until they eventually occur. Explain to your child that feeling these emotions are normal and that they should not feel afraid of it. Instead, encourage your child to take control of these emotions and "survive." This helps to create strength to cope. You need to emphasize that once your child takes charge of these emotions, it will be easier for them to think more logically despite being angry.

4. Try to keep the focus on your child and not you.

You may feel hesitant to offer your personal experience with a similar issue. Instead, just listen and offer your support if your kids ask for it. Sometimes your child simply needs a shoulder to cry on, or sometimes they may approach you to help them out of a situation. Anticipating their needs or even verbalizing what they need in the current situation is an excellent strategy to make sure you keep the focus on your child and help them feel seen during difficult times.

Kids sometimes do not like it when their parents meddle with their personal affairs. So, if the issue is not pressing enough to cause concern, let your child handle it. Then, when your child seeks you for help, then that is the time that you act.

5. Children feel better when they feel understood.

Children will accept more than merely being offered a solution. Remember that kids can think on their own as well. Sometimes kids would rather have you not provide a solution for their problem but understand them and know where they are coming from, rather than you offering a solution. It's helpful to try and relate to your child's situation and recall how you might have felt at that age. Recall yourself ever facing the same situation or consider how you might have reacted. Be open and honest with your children when you try to understand them. Sometimes you may not even know how they feel but being able to empathize and show compassion is so important.

Do not alienate yourself from the problem, but not be too meddlesome either. Listen to what your child has to say. Put yourself on his/her shoe and view the situation from their perspective. That will be a much better "solution" you can offer to your child.

6. Timing is everything.

After a long day at school, children need to rest and refresh their batteries.

There is no right time to have deep conversations and a conversation that addresses problems (this is also the moment that monosyllables respond to parents!).

Instead, why not schedule a specific time at home for a few minutes of chat? Scheduling a type gives your children a chance to prepare themselves, and the same goes for parents as well.

This could be before bed, after they cool down, or maybe after "working time" or "meetings." It is smart to try to relax them — maybe even over tea/coffee, hot cocoa, or a sweet treat! Get your children comfortable and let them know that they can divulge anything they want without fear of reper-

PROBLEM HANDLING FOR CHILDREN | 99

cussions. This is a time for them to express what has been weighing heavily on them, or negatively impacting them. It may even only be a chance to share the positive things that have been affecting their lives. Whatever they choose to talk about, it is your chance to get a deeper understanding of your child.

When you approach your children to engage in a heart-to-heart conservation, you need them in a time where they are not busy, relaxed, and ready to open. Do not suddenly spring a conversation with them on deep or heavy topics when they are not mentally prepared or anticipating it. But once you do start with the deep conversations, you can make this a routine either daily or weekly. It is even better if you have a scheduled daily "check-up" talk and a weekly "deep" talk.

7. Encourage your child to think, plan, and reassess before acting.

You help them learn an essential life skill by showing them that resolving problems is not an immediate answer but a continuous process. You must make your child understand that solving real-life problems is not like problems solved at school, where you only must perform a certain step, and you will already get the answer. Emphasize to your child that problems in life are more complicated than they think. They themselves are a process, and that as you look for ways to solve them, you need to think, plan, and reassess things before you can find the best solution.

Furthermore, this can encourage children to be more result-oriented where they begin assessing their abilities through their performance, rather than the achievement at the end. This is a great way to get your kids to strive to perform better and look at themselves critically as they follow through with their plans.

You can also let your child read newspapers or chat with friends for experience in sharing their opinions and listening to other people. They will also benefit from picking up views in a newspaper or chatting to others as they learn about the diversity that exists around us.

8. Asking for help is a sign of strength, not weakness.

Kids sometimes think that asking for help from others, especially their parents, is a sign of weakness. You need to make your kids understand that asking for help is not a weakness but a strength. Remember this and instil this in the mind of your kid before your kid accepts it!

But you also must emphasize that asking for help every time is also not a good practice. Your kid should know when to ask for help and when to rely on him/herself. With this, you will be able to develop a sense of independence in your child and a sense of confidence in their abilities to solve problems on their own or seek help from others.

9. Applaud your child's strengths and focus on positive outcomes.

Your child needs positive reinforcement and not just constant reminders and notifications of their misdemeanours. This is where parents have to find a suitable medium between disciplining their children and focusing on their good behaviour. When you notice that your child has done something right or accomplished a task, you must acknowledge that.

Tell them you are proud of their contributions to coping with stringent circumstances. You will soon notice that your child will take an even more active role in helping you.

Be specific and descriptive with your words as effusive positive words can come off disingenuous or insincere as the more general it is, the less likely it is to be relevant to your child. ("I'm an angel for sharing my toys? What about not doing homework last night?") Children can sometimes perceive the disingenuous praise and instead use it to reflect on their behaviour and consider how they acted contrary to the praise when you use sweeping terms for praise.

10. Encourage your child to have a support network.

Emphasize to your child that being alone in dealing with problems is not good. You need to make your child understand the importance of keeping the right friends and being open to family. Bottling up feelings and pent up anger can lead to disastrous results.

As a parent, you can provide a safe space for your kids to share their feelings and express anything that has had a negative impact on their mental health. Be a non-judgmental listener and provide support when they need it. Support comes in plenty of forms, sometimes it means being a shoulder to cry on, or sometimes it means being more proactive and providing the solution outright to them. Regardless of the issue and its scope, being present for your child is crucial for their development.

At the same time, your child can also have other people involved in their support system to ground them and help them navigate through life. This can be anyone your child will feel comfortable to approach and divulge their feelings with. Many adults, family members and peers can become involved in their support system. As long as your child does not feel alone or like an outcast or afterthought, you are already taking steps in the right direction.

Remember that every parenting (family) journey is different, and a destination is reached in several ways. So, do not limit your options to yourself. If others can help your child, then include them. As much as parents cling onto the idea of their children being dependent on them for a very long time, they eventually have to let go of this notion and allow their children to peacefully make their own social connections and build trust with other people who may enter into their lives.

PRACTICE SOLVING PROBLEMS

Do not rush to fix your child's issues for him if difficulties occur. Help him go over the problem-solving phase instead. Provide advice when he needs support, but empower him to fix things himself.

If he cannot find a way, move in to make him learn of available options. The key is to avoid telling him what to do immediately because you want your children to be able to process a new situation and figure out the best course of action independently.

You need to serve as the guide for your child and not the problem-solver. If you solve every single problem your child experiences, how will they learn and grow? So, give your child the chance to think on their own and look for solutions to their problems. But welcome them as well if they take the initiative to ask for your help. Encourage different ways to approach solutions and be a source for your child to bounce their ideas off of. You can still provide advice for your child, but encourage them to voice what they think and what they feel compelled to do in the situation.

Using a problem-solving strategy when you experience behavioural problems:

Solving problems that involve your child can be difficult. That is why you need to have a solid strategy on how to deal with them.

For example, you can sit down with your child and say, "It was challenging to get your homework done lately. Let us solve it together."

You will also have to deal with their misbehaviour, and the same thing applies. You need to be sure that you have invested in finding a solution so that your kids can do better next time.

8

HOW TO RAISE YOUR TYPE OF CHILD

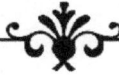

❦

One of the mistakes that parents often commit when raising their children is that they do not consider what type of child they have. A disciplinary action that is effective for one child may not be as effective for another child.

That is because children varied in their personalities and thought processes. Some children are more sensitive than others. Some are more difficult than others. In comparison, some are clever and need less supervision.

If you want to raise your child well, you need to consider the things that make your child unique: their learning styles, their habits, their personality, etc. No two children are the same, and as such, no single parenting method is going to apply effectively to every child. Your children do not fall into a category but instead may inhibit certain characteristics. Ultimately, children are a mix of all of the following "types". Some children may be more emotional than others. The same be said about stubborn or strong-willed children. Finding the right parenting style is part of the journey of parenthood that must be faced. Mothers and fathers can then apply the necessary disciplinary actions according to their child's needs.

RAISING AN EMOTIONAL CHILD

One of the main problems with emotional children is that they do not have a full grasp of their emotions. They can cry for the littlest things. It does not also help that many parents have negative reactions when they see their child crying, especially in public. This should not be. If your child is emotional, here are some tips that you can apply:

Crying is not necessarily a weakness. It is usual for children to cry, but some parents become embarrassed if their child cries in public. For example, a father may see his child crying over fallen ice cream. The father cringes from the scene and immediately scolds the child or takes the child away. The same thing may happen for a mother who sees her daughter crying because she lost.

If your child is emotional, it does not mean that your child is weak. They simply do not have control of their emotions yet. That is why, as parents, it is your role to help your child recognize their emotions and understand how to control them.

Put a name on the emotion. Sometimes a child may cry but may not fully understand why they are really crying. You must put a name on the emotion they are feeling. For example, you can say, "You are crying because you are sad that you lost." You can name your emotions as well so that the child can relate to how you feel. You can say, "I am sad that you did not do your homework today."

You can drill on this by watching movies or reading books and asking the child how the characters are feeling. It will help them associate the names of emotions with how they look and feel.

Differentiate feelings and behaviour. You must tell your child that they can feel all those emotions, but they can decide on how to respond to those emotions. You need to emphasize that there are certain behaviours more appropriate for a certain emotion. For example, you can say, "It is okay to be angry, but you cannot hit anyone because of it." Or, "It is okay to cry, but you cannot throw a tantrum."

Discipline the behaviour, not the emotions. Inform your child that whatever emotions they feel, it is normal, but once they behave inappropriate in response to those emotions, then there are consequences. For example, you can say, "I will be taking your toys for a day because you were screaming when you cried, and it is not a good behaviour." Allow your children to express their emotions in an appropriate way, rather than encouraging them to suppress them.

Do not minimize a child's emotions. One mistake that many parents commit is underestimating their child's feelings. For example, some parents will tell their child to stop crying because the problem is not a crying matter. This is wrong. You need to validate what and how your child feels so they can better understand. For example, you can say, "You are mad because I did not buy you ice cream. I also get mad when I do not get what I want too. But you should not cry about it because there is still next time, or another day called tomorrow."

Teach emotion regulation. You need to teach your child how they can regulate and manage their emotions and keep them under control. Here are some skills you can teach:

1. Take a quiet moment to process their emotions.
2. Try some deep breathing exercising to regulate your heart and breathing.
3. Count from 1 to 10.
4. Closing their eyes and relax.
5. Create a kit to cheer up.
6. Do a hobby to boost mood.

RAISING AN EMPATHIC CHILD

Empathic kids understand the feelings of others and know how to deal with their own emotions and the emotions of others. If you want your child to develop empathy, then here are some tips:

Help your child understand their own feelings. Empathic people understand the feelings of others because they have a full understanding of their feelings. You need to help your child make sense of their emotions first. Explain what positive and negative emotions are and what your child can do in response to them.

Do not hide the truth. Some parents shield their children from the harsh realities of the world, which downgrades the importance of these realities. This can give the wrong impression to the child that these issues do not matter. Talk about these issues (e.g., bullying, school shootings, allergies, the effect of coronavirus, global crisis) with your child and make them understand their importance. Even if they do not thoroughly understand them yet, at least they will have an idea.

A demonstration is a good option. If you want your child to be empathic, then you have to be empathic yourself. Stay calm in stressful situations. Process your emotions first before reacting immediately. Model this to your child.

Take action and show kindness. Actions speak louder than words. Model kind behaviour if you want your children to do the same. Take a moment of your day to slow down and show kindness to others. Any small act will do as ultimately, and your children are always observing how you treat others and will absorb the same behaviours and habits. Help an elderly cross the street. Help the neighbour with a chore. How you display your capacity for compassion can really leave a mark on your children. These are little things that when you show your child, they will still realize the importance of being kind.

RAISING A STRONG-WILLED CHILD

Raising a strong-willed child is probably one of the greatest challenges of a parent. That is because, unlike other children, strong-willed children tend to be more stubborn and courageous enough to defy their parents, especially if they have their own viewpoints against a particular matter. Therefore, most parents who have strong-willed children end up in a power-struggle against their own kids. If you are experiencing the same problem with your child, then here are some tips you can follow:

Teach through experience. Strong-willed children learn best through experience. That is why they do not easily believe what you say when they do not experience it themselves. For example, when you tell your child not to touch the stove because it is hot, they will confirm if it is hot before they believe you. Use that to your advantage. When you discipline your child, it is best if they experience the effect first, unless there is a risk for serious injury.

Give them independence. It is better if you give your child to be independent. Instead of nagging them to do things, give them reminders instead. For example, instead of telling a child to do their homework and not play, you can say, "Before playing, what do you need to do?" This way, you are not directly telling them what to do but reminding them by asking the question.

Do not give orders. Like giving them independence, give your child choices instead of orders. It affords them the autonomy that they deserve. For example, you need to ask your child to do some chores, but they are playing. You can say, "You need to pause your playing for a moment and help me with the trash. Do you want to help me now and still have a chance to play before bed? Or do you want to continue playing and help me with the trash later. But it's going to be too dark outside later on." Being a figure of authority in a child's life does not mean that every order you demand should be met.

Implement routines. To avoid having to constantly wrestle power from your child and being the bad guy for forcing them, you need to set up a routine and ground rules. Children thrive on a routine because it sets their days up in an organized way so that they know what to expect and aren't overwhelmed by the possibilities. You must make sure that your child agrees to them as well. That way, when your child commits something that breaks the rules, you must remind them that they agreed to the routine and the rules beforehand, including the consequences.

Listen to what your child has to say. Your child has their own views and opinions on things. You must listen to what they say. Even when you know they are wrong, give them a chance to share why they think are right. By listening carefully, will you understand why your child is opposing you or acting in a certain way? This will also help you see the issue from their point of view.

Respect your children. As you expect your children to respect you, the same goes vice versa. Children are human beings and deserve respect as they navigate through life. Since your child has strong views on things, you must respect that. Make them understand your views by talking about it to them. In the same way, discuss their views with them as well. This will help both you and your child, where each of you is coming from regarding the problem. These are opportune moments to teach your child that people are always going to have a different perspective, and not everyone will agree with them.

FINAL THOUGHTS

Raising a child is never easy. Parenthood is not something that is taught in schools, and the best way to truly get a good grasp on being a parent is through experience. You learn as you go along and experience what it is like to raise a child. However, one thing that you should really put effort into understanding is how to raise your child is their nature. Do not lump your child together with your friend's child. All children are incredibly different and unique from each other and have been shaped by different things in their lives. Your disciplinary methods must match the type of child that you have. Only then will you be able to observe positive changes in their behaviours.

LEAVE A REVIEW!

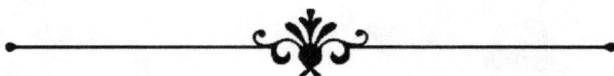

After reading this book, please feel free to leave a review based on your findings and how useful the guide was to you. I would be incredibly thankful if you could take 60 seconds to write a brief review on Amazon, even if it's just a few sentences!

CONCLUSION

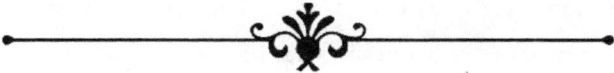

Discipline is about behaviour modification, not about punishing kids. Discipline encourages kids to develop self-discipline and helps them become adults who are mentally and socially mature. Many efficient approaches can help parents teach their children and direct them, and certain types of discipline will remain controversial.

As you try to instil good habits and good behaviour within your children, parents will sometimes come across moments of anxiety as they question their capabilities and their methods. This is something that parents around the world have experienced for generations. Being a good parent is a Herculean task, but by no means is it impossible. Having faith and trusting in your own capabilities to love and nourish your children comes first to being a good parent. From this vantage point, as you discipline your children and walk them through life, you will be bound to make mistakes but know that children are resilient in their own way. Be vulnerable with your children and respect them so that you realize when it is time to apologize to them.

Always remember that there is no one right way to train a child. Do your best, trust God to help you, and enjoy the company of the little ones in your life.

OTHER BOOKS YOU'LL LOVE!

CLICK ON THE BOOKS

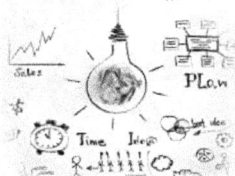

LIFE STRATEGIES
FOR
TEENAGERS

Positive Parenting, Tips and Understanding Teens for Better Communication and a Happy Family

BUKKY EKINE-OGUNLANA

Link to Book

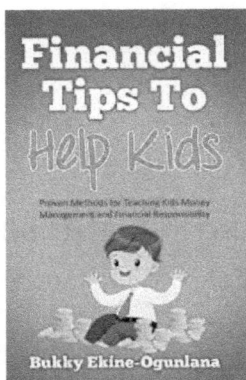

Link to Book

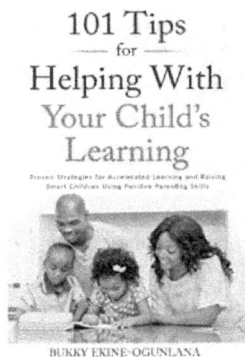

Link to Book

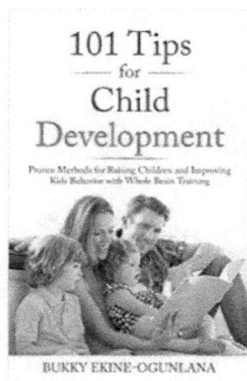

Link to Book

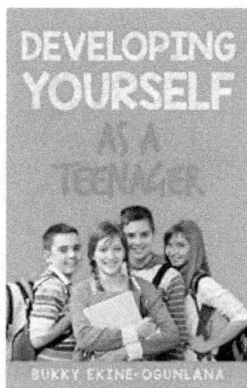

Link to Book

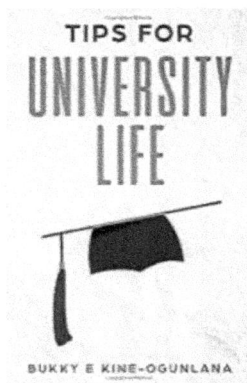

Link to Book

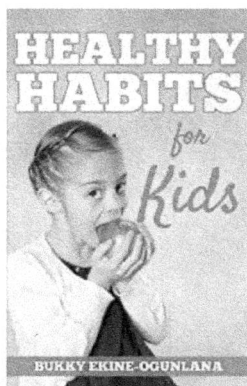

Link to Book

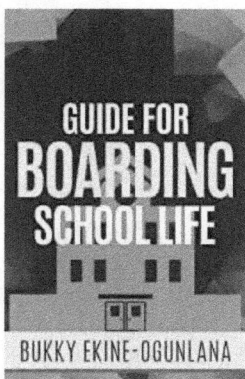

Link to Book

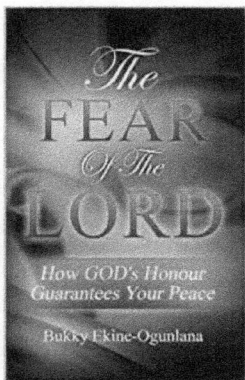

Link to Book

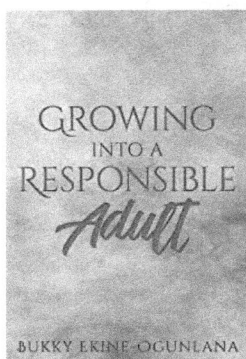

Link to Book

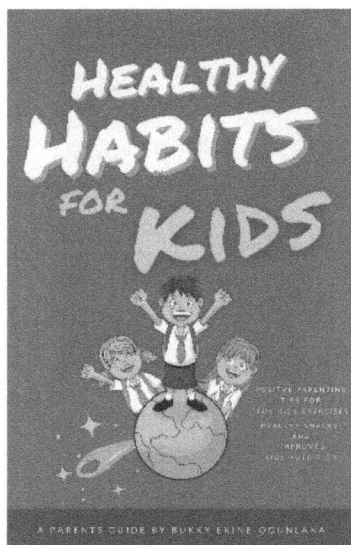

Link to Book

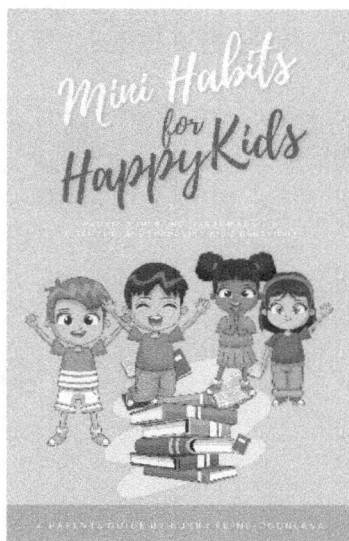

Link to Book

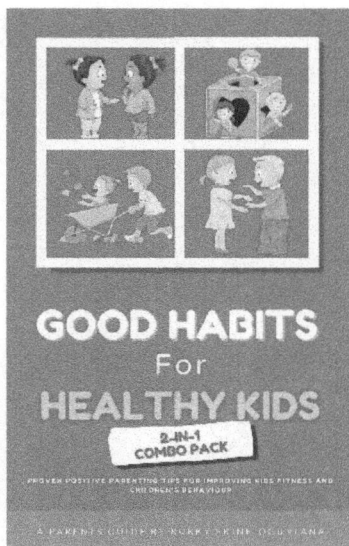

Link to Book

REFERENCES

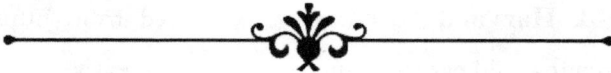

Tips for Parents: Teaching Discipline to Your Children. Retrieved from https://preventchildabuse.org/resource/tips-for-parents-teaching-discipline-to-your-children/

School Administrator's Top 10 Discipline Tips All Parents Should Know. Retrieved from http://www.parent-institute.com/reports-for-delivery/10-Discipline-Tips-Report.pdf

Discipline (0 – 12 years). Retrieved from https://www.education.sa.gov.au/sites/default/files/parentingsa/peg2.pdf?v=1489727260

Discipline in the Early Years. Retrieved from http://learnatcstreet.org/data/documents/Child-Discipline.pdf

How to Discipline Toddlers by Rachel Ehmke. Retrieved from https://childmind.org/article/how-discipline-toddlers/

Three Principles to Improve Outcomes for Children and Families by Center on the Developing Child, Harvard University. Retrieved from https://developingchild.harvard.edu/resources/three-early-childhood-development-principles-improve-child-family-outcomes/

Effective discipline for children. (2004). *Pediatrics& child health*, *9*(1), 37–50. Retrieved from https://doi.org/10.1093/pch/9.1.37

Discipline and Guiding Behaviour: **Babies and Children**. Retrieved from https://raisingchildren.net.au/toddlers/behaviour/discipline/discipline-strategies#choosing-an-approach-to-discipline-nav-title

Positive Discipline: A Guide for Parents. Retrieved from http://pcit-toddlers.org/resources/umn-positive-discipline-a-guide-for-parents.pdf

Great Habits for Kids to Have Early in Life. Retrieved from https://afgfamily.com/blog/news/8-great-habits-for-kids-to-have-early-in-life/

https://parenting.firstcry.com/articles/12-habits-of-parents-who-are-raising-successful-children/

An age-by-age guide to disciplining your kid. Retrieved from https://www.todaysparent.com/kids/preschool/disciplining-children-age-by-age-guide/

Parents, Kids, and Discipline. Retrieved from https://www.webmd.com/parenting/guide/discipline-tactics

God made you be creative. Retrieved from https://douglastalks.com/god-made-you-to-be-creative-a-lesson-about-creativity-for-kids/

Ways to Boost Child's Creative Thinking. Retrieved from https://ezplaytoys.com/blogs/blog/creativity-for-kids-15-ways-to-boost-childs-creative-thinking

How to Help an Overly Emotional Child Cope with Their Feelings. Retrieved from https://www.verywellfamily.com/how-to-help-an-overly-emotional-child-4157594

4 Ways to Raise an Empathic Child. Retrieved from https://www.positiveparentingsolutions.com/parenting/4-ways-to-raise-an-empathy-rich-child

The strong-willed child: 11 ways to turn power struggles into cooperation. Retrieved from https://

www.mother.ly/child/11-tips-for-parenting-your-strong-willed-child/5-avoid-power-struggles-by-using-routines-and-rules

Like us on https://www.facebook.com/tcecpublishing/

http://www.thechildrenseducationcentre.co.uk/specialoffer